It is Possible to Eat well, get
SLIMMER
and
HEALTHIER,
I did it you can do it too.
BOOK BY
BLESSED WOWPLUS
HEALTH NUTRIONIST

In today's society, there is a growing concern about body weight and its impact on overall health. While many factors contribute to weight gain or loss, the role of diet is undeniable. What we eat has a direct impact on our body weight, and understanding the relationship between the two is crucial for achieving optimal health and well-being.

This book aims to explore the complex interplay between eating and body weight. We will examine how different types of food affect our metabolism, energy balance, and fat storage, as well as the hormonal and psychological factors that influence our eating behaviors.

Through a comprehensive review of the scientific literature and practical examples, we will debunk common myths and misconceptions about weight loss and gain, and provide evidence-based strategies for achieving and maintaining a healthy weight.

Whether you are struggling with weight management or simply interested in learning more about the science of nutrition, this book offers a valuable resource for understanding the impact of diet on body weight and overall health.

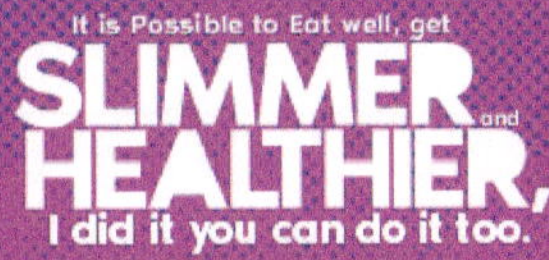

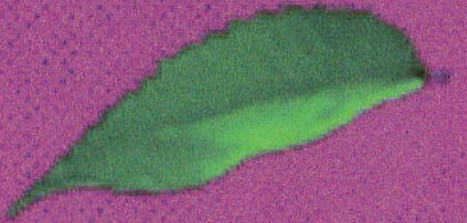

CHAPTER 1

The importance of a balanced and nutritious diet for overall health and well-being

I firmly believe that it is possible to eat well, get slimmer, and healthier at the same time. The key to achieving this goal is to adopt a balanced and sustainable approach to nutrition that focuses on nourishing the body with nutrient-dense whole foods while avoiding processed and refined foods that can lead to weight gain and poor health.

One of the most important steps to achieving optimal health is to consume a wide variety of nutrient-dense foods, including fruits, vegetables, whole grains, lean proteins, and healthy fats. These foods are packed with essential vitamins, minerals, and antioxidants that can support a healthy metabolism, improve immune function, and reduce the risk of chronic disease.

In addition to focusing on whole foods, it is also essential to pay attention to portion sizes and meal frequency. Consuming smaller, more frequent meals throughout the day can help to keep blood sugar levels stable, reduce cravings, and promote satiety. It is also important to avoid skipping meals or restricting calories too severely, as this can slow down the metabolism and make weight loss more difficult.

Another key factor in achieving optimal health is to stay hydrated by drinking plenty of water throughout the day. Water is essential for maintaining healthy digestion, regulating body temperature, and flushing toxins from the body. It can also help to reduce cravings and promote feelings of fullness, which can help to prevent overeating.

Maintaining a healthy weight is crucial for preventing chronic diseases and enhancing overall well-being. While exercise is an important component of weight loss, a healthy diet is equally essential. This study aims to investigate the relationship between healthy eating and weight loss by examining the effects of a balanced diet on metabolism, digestion, chronic disease risk, and overall health

Finally, it is important to engage in regular physical activity to support overall health and wellness. Exercise can help to burn calories, increase muscle mass, improve cardiovascular health, and reduce stress levels. By combining a balanced and nutritious diet with regular exercise, it is possible to achieve a healthy weight, reduce the risk of chronic disease, and feel great both inside and out.

what are the signs people with weight issues face:

People with weight issues may experience a variety of signs and symptoms related to their weight. Here are some common signs people with weight issues may face:

Increased body fat: One of the most obvious signs of weight issues is increased body fat. People who are overweight or obese often carry excess fat around their midsection, hips, and thighs.

Difficulty losing weight: People with weight issues may find it difficult to lose weight, even when they are following a healthy diet and exercising regularly. This can be due to a variety of factors, including metabolic issues, hormone imbalances, or underlying health conditions.

Low energy levels: Carrying excess weight can put a strain on the body and lead to low energy levels. People with weight issues may feel tired or fatigued even after getting enough sleep.

Joint pain: Carrying excess weight can also put extra strain on the joints, leading to joint pain and stiffness. This can make it difficult to engage in physical activity, which can exacerbate weight issues.

Increased risk of chronic disease: Being overweight or obese can increase the risk of a variety of chronic health conditions, including type 2 diabetes, heart disease, and certain types of cancer.

Poor sleep quality: People with weight issues may also experience poor sleep quality, including difficulty falling asleep or staying asleep. This can be due to a variety of factors, including sleep apnea and other breathing disorders.

There are many good food ideas that can help you get slimmer and healthier. Here are some examples:

Lean Protein: Including lean protein sources like chicken, fish, tofu, and beans in your diet can help you feel full and satisfied for longer periods. This can help you avoid overeating and make it easier to maintain a calorie deficit, which is essential for weight loss.

Vegetables and Fruits: Vegetables and fruits are high in fiber, vitamins, and minerals that are essential for good health. They are also low in calories, so including plenty of these foods in your diet can help you feel full and satisfied without consuming too many calories.

Whole Grains: Whole grains like brown rice, quinoa, and whole-wheat bread are high in fiber, which can help you feel full and satisfied. They are also more nutritious than refined grains, which have been stripped of many essential nutrients.

Healthy Fats: Healthy fats like avocados, nuts, and olive oil can help you feel full and satisfied while also providing important nutrients for your body. They are also essential for good health, as they can help reduce inflammation and lower the risk of heart disease.

Water: Drinking plenty of water throughout the day can help you feel full and satisfied, which can help you avoid overeating. It can also help keep you hydrated, which is important for good health.

Overall, incorporating these healthy food ideas into your diet can help you get slimmer and healthier by providing your body with essential nutrients while also helping you maintain a calorie deficit for weight loss.

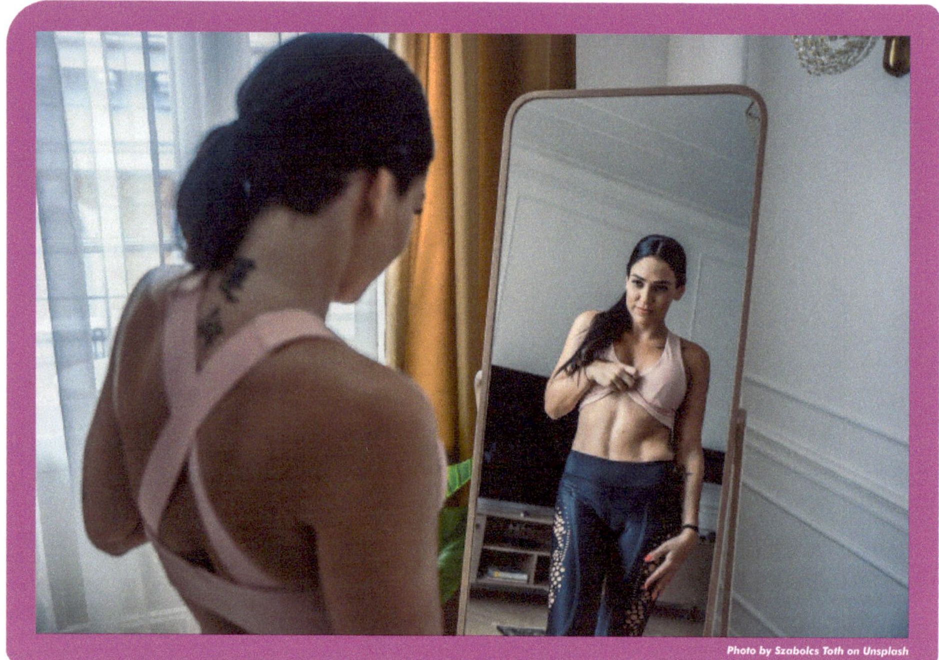

Photo by Szabolcs Toth on Unsplash

In conclusion

it is absolutely possible to eat well, get slimmer, and improve overall health at the same time. By adopting a balanced and sustainable approach to nutrition, staying hydrated, and engaging in regular physical activity, anyone can achieve their health and wellness goals and enjoy a happier, healthier life.

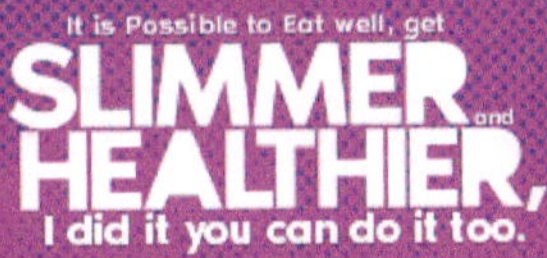

CHAPTER 2

The benefits of eating a variety of fruits, vegetables, whole grains, and lean proteins

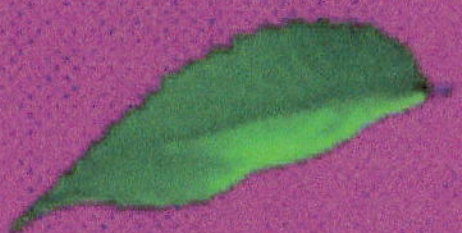

A balanced and nutritious diet is crucial for overall health and well-being. It provides the body with the essential nutrients it needs to function properly, maintain optimal health, and prevent chronic diseases. Fruits are an important part of a healthy and balanced diet, providing essential nutrients such as vitamins, minerals, fiber, and antioxidants. While eating fruits in general is beneficial to health, consuming a variety of fruits is equally important.

This chapter aims to investigate the health benefits of eating a variety of fruits and the impact it has on reducing the risk of chronic diseases. Not eating fruits can lead to various diseases, including:

Cardiovascular disease: Fruits are a rich source of antioxidants and fiber, which have been linked to a reduced risk of cardiovascular disease. Not consuming enough fruits can increase the risk of developing heart disease, stroke, and other cardiovascular conditions.

Type 2 diabetes: A diet low in fruits and high in refined carbohydrates and processed foods has been associated with an increased risk of developing type 2 diabetes. Fruits contain natural sugars that can help regulate blood sugar levels and prevent insulin resistance.

Cancer: Eating a variety of fruits has been linked to a reduced risk of certain types of cancer, including lung, colon, and breast cancer. Fruits contain phytonutrients and antioxidants that can help protect cells from damage and prevent the development of cancer cells.

Digestive disorders: Fruits are a good source of fiber, which is important for maintaining digestive health. Not consuming enough fruits can lead to constipation, bloating, and other digestive disorders.

Nutrient deficiencies: Fruits are a rich source of vitamins and minerals, including vitamin C, potassium, and folate. Not consuming enough fruits can lead to nutrient deficiencies, which can weaken the immune system, increase the risk of infections, and impair cognitive function.

In summary, not eating enough fruits can have serious consequences for overall health and increase the risk of developing various chronic diseases. It is important to incorporate a variety of fruits into the diet to ensure optimal health and well-being.

Whole grains are an essential component of a healthy and balanced diet. They are rich in fiber, vitamins, minerals, and antioxidants that provide numerous health benefits. Here are some of the key nutrient values and health benefits of whole grains:

Nutrient Values:

Fiber: Whole grains are an excellent source of dietary fiber, which helps to promote healthy digestion, prevent constipation, and reduce the risk of developing digestive disorders such as diverticulitis and irritable bowel syndrome.

Vitamins: Whole grains are rich in vitamins such as vitamin B and E, which are important for maintaining healthy skin, eyes, and immune system function.

Minerals: Whole grains are a good source of essential minerals such as iron, magnesium, and selenium, which are important for maintaining healthy bones, teeth, and overall body function.

Antioxidants: Whole grains contain antioxidants such as phenolic acids and flavonoids, which help to protect the body against oxidative stress and reduce the risk of chronic diseases such as heart disease, cancer, and Alzheimer's disease.

Health Benefits:

Reducing the risk of chronic diseases: Whole grains have been shown to reduce the risk of chronic diseases such as heart disease, stroke, type 2 diabetes, and certain types of cancer. The high fiber content of whole grains can help to lower cholesterol levels and regulate blood sugar levels, reducing the risk of heart disease and type 2 diabetes.

Promoting weight management: Whole grains are more filling than refined grains, which can help to promote feelings of fullness and reduce overall calorie intake. This can be beneficial for weight management and reducing the risk of obesity.

Improving gut health: The fiber content of whole grains helps to promote healthy gut bacteria, which can improve digestive health and reduce the risk of digestive disorders such as constipation, diarrhea, and inflammatory bowel disease.

Supporting cognitive function: Whole grains contain nutrients such as vitamin E and selenium, which have been linked to improved cognitive function and a reduced risk of cognitive decline and dementia.

Here are some of the key reasons why a balanced and nutritious diet is so important:

Provides essential nutrients: A balanced and nutritious diet includes a variety of whole foods that are rich in essential nutrients such as vitamins, minerals, fiber, and antioxidants. These nutrients are important for maintaining healthy body functions and preventing nutrient deficiencies that can lead to health problems.

Supports healthy digestion: A diet that includes plenty of fiber-rich fruits, vegetables, whole grains, and legumes can support healthy digestion and prevent digestive issues such as constipation and diarrhea.

Maintains healthy weight: A balanced and nutritious diet can help maintain a healthy weight, which is important for preventing chronic diseases such as heart disease, type 2 diabetes, and certain types of cancer.

Reduces the risk of chronic diseases: A diet that is high in fruits, vegetables, whole grains, lean proteins, and healthy fats can help reduce the risk of chronic diseases such as heart disease, stroke, and certain types of cancer.

Boosts immune function: A diet that is rich in nutrients can help support a healthy immune system, which is important for preventing infections and illnesses.

Improves energy levels: Eating a balanced and nutritious diet can help improve energy levels, which can help increase productivity and improve overall quality of life.

Promotes mental health: A healthy diet can also have a positive impact on mental health, reducing the risk of depression and anxiety and improving overall mood and well-being.

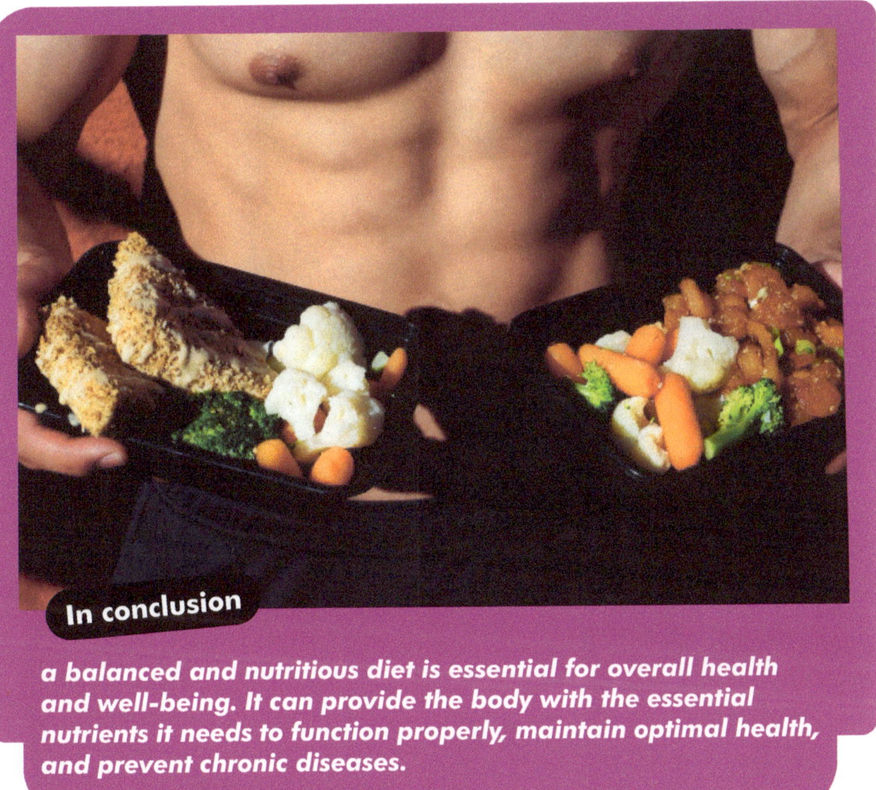

a balanced and nutritious diet is essential for overall health and well-being. It can provide the body with the essential nutrients it needs to function properly, maintain optimal health, and prevent chronic diseases.

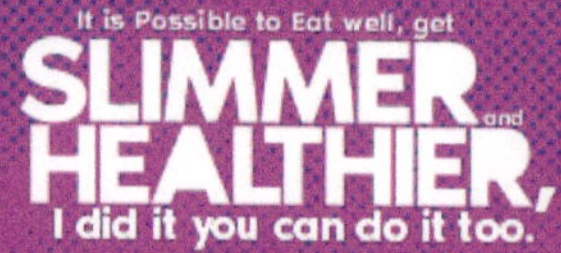

CHAPTER 3

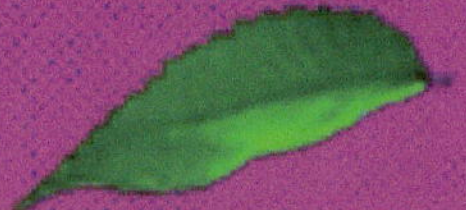

The role of portion control and mindful eating in weight management

Portion control plays a crucial role in weight loss because it helps to manage calorie intake. When you eat more calories than your body burns, the excess calories are stored as fat, leading to weight gain. By controlling your portion sizes, you can reduce your calorie intake and create a calorie deficit, which can help you lose weight.

Advantages of portion control for weight loss:

Helps you stay within your calorie goals: Portion control helps you manage your calorie intake by ensuring that you don't overeat or eat more than what your body needs.

Reduces the risk of overeating: By eating smaller portions, you're less likely to feel too full and have the urge to continue eating, which can lead to overeating.

Encourages mindful eating: When you focus on portion control, you're more likely to pay attention to your hunger and fullness cues, leading to more mindful eating habits.

Allows you to enjoy a variety of foods: By controlling your portions, you can still enjoy your favorite foods in moderation without having to give them up completely.

Disadvantages of portion control for weight loss:

Can be difficult to stick to: Portion control requires discipline and may be challenging to follow, especially when you're eating out or in social settings.

May be time-consuming: Measuring and weighing your food to ensure you're eating the right portion size can be time-consuming, which may not be practical for everyone.

May not work for everyone: Portion control may not be effective for everyone, as some people may need to follow more structured diets or work with a nutritionist to achieve their weight loss goals.

Overall, portion control can be an effective tool for weight loss, but it's important to find a balance that works for you and your lifestyle. It's also essential to focus on making sustainable lifestyle changes to maintain a healthy weight in the long term.

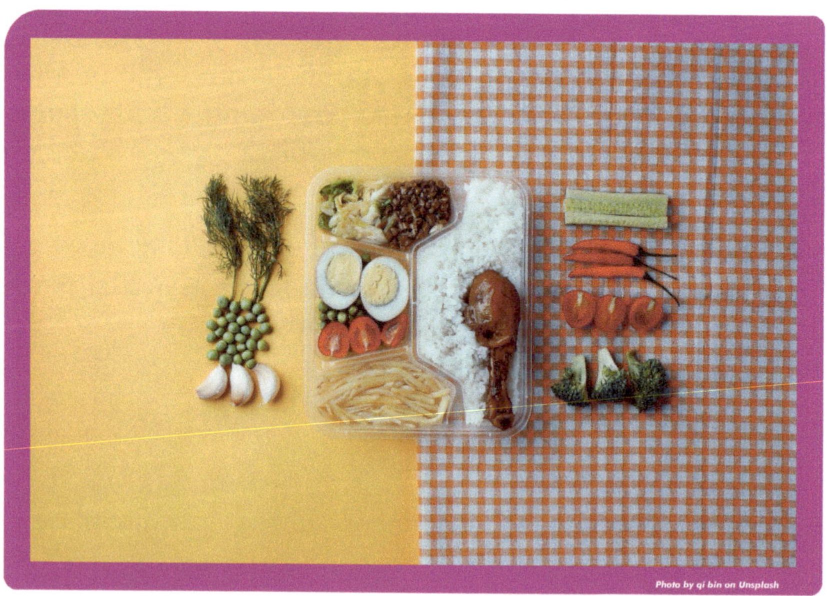

Photo by qi bin on Unsplash

It is Possible to Eat well, Get slimmer and healthier, I did it you can do it too.

How can you identify the amount of calories you eat daily:

There are several ways to identify the amount of calories you eat daily:

Use a food diary: Keeping a food diary or using a food tracking app can help you track what you eat and estimate the number of calories you consume daily.

Read nutrition labels: Most packaged foods have nutrition labels that provide information about the number of calories per serving. Use this information to calculate the total number of calories you consume.

Use a kitchen scale: Weighing your food with a kitchen scale can help you accurately measure the amount you eat and calculate the calories.

Use an online calorie calculator: There are many online calorie calculators that can help you estimate the number of calories you consume daily based on your height, weight, age, and activity level.

It's important to note that these methods provide estimates and may not be 100% accurate. However, by consistently tracking your calorie intake, you can get a better idea of how many calories you consume daily and make adjustments to meet your weight loss or maintenance goals.

Weight management myths and facts:

Weight management is an essential aspect of maintaining a healthy lifestyle. Unfortunately, there are many myths and misconceptions surrounding weight management that can make it challenging to achieve your goals. Here are some common weight management myths and facts:

Myth: You can lose weight quickly and easily with fad diets or weight loss supplements.

Fact: Fad diets and weight loss supplements are often ineffective in the long term and can even be harmful to your health. Sustainable weight loss requires a balanced diet, regular exercise, and healthy lifestyle habits.

Myth: Carbs are bad for weight loss.

Fact: Carbs are an essential source of energy and should be included in a balanced diet. However, it's important to choose complex carbs like whole grains, fruits, and vegetables, instead of simple carbs like refined sugars.

Myth: Skipping meals can help you lose weight.

Fact: Skipping meals can lead to overeating later in the day and can slow down your metabolism, making it harder to lose weight. It's better to eat regular, balanced meals throughout the day to maintain a healthy metabolism.

Myth: Fat-free or low-fat foods are always a healthy choice.

Fact: Many fat-free or low-fat foods are high in sugar and other unhealthy additives to compensate for the lack of fat. It's important to read nutrition labels and choose whole, nutrient-dense foods instead of highly processed alternatives.

Myth: Exercise is the most important factor for weight loss.

Fact: Exercise is crucial for overall health and can support weight loss, but diet and lifestyle habits also play a significant role in weight management. It's essential to adopt a balanced approach to diet, exercise, and lifestyle changes for sustainable weight loss.

In conclusion

it's important to be aware of weight management myths and seek accurate information from credible sources. By adopting a balanced approach to diet, exercise, and lifestyle habits, you can achieve your weight management goals and maintain a healthy lifestyle.

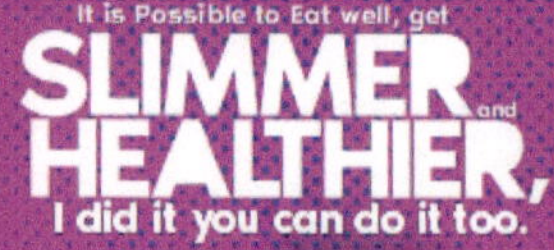

CHAPTER 4

The potential benefits of reducing or eliminating processed and unhealthy foods from the diet

Processed foods can be harmful to the human body in several ways, and they can contribute to weight gain and obesity.

One of the primary concerns with processed foods is that they are often high in calories, unhealthy fats, sugars, and salt. These ingredients can lead to weight gain, especially when consumed in excess.

Additionally, many processed foods lack essential nutrients that the body needs to function properly. For example, many processed foods are stripped of fiber, which is essential for maintaining healthy digestion and feeling full and satisfied after eating.

Processed foods are also often treated with chemicals and additives that can be harmful to the body, such as preservatives, artificial colors and flavors, and high-fructose corn syrup. These additives can contribute to inflammation in the body, which can lead to a host of health problems, including weight gain, type 2 diabetes, and heart disease.

Overall, while some processed foods can be part of a healthy diet in moderation, consuming too many processed foods can have negative effects on the body and contribute to weight gain and other health problems. It's generally recommended to focus on whole, unprocessed foods whenever possible for optimal health and weight management.

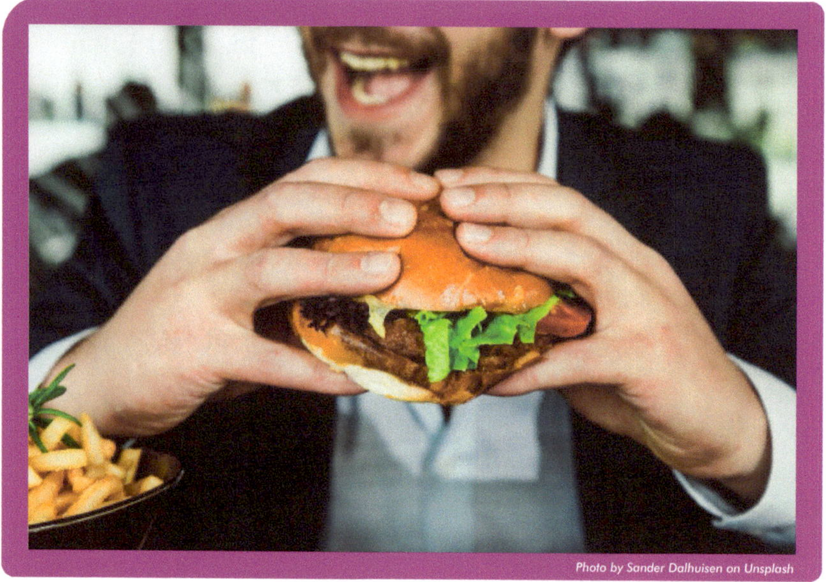

Photo by Sander Dalhuisen on Unsplash

Unhealthy foods are those that are high in calories, unhealthy fats, added sugars, and/or refined carbohydrates. Consuming these types of foods regularly can lead to weight gain and other negative health consequences. Here's a closer look at the process, advantages, and disadvantages of consuming unhealthy foods:

Process:

When you consume unhealthy foods, your body breaks them down into glucose (sugar), which enters your bloodstream and provides energy to your cells. However, when you consume more calories than your body needs, the excess glucose is converted into fat and stored in adipose tissue throughout your body. Over time, consuming too many unhealthy foods can lead to a buildup of excess body fat and weight gain.

Advantages:

There are not many advantages to consuming unhealthy foods regularly. However, some people may find that consuming these types of foods in moderation can provide a temporary boost in mood or energy. Additionally, some unhealthy foods may contain certain nutrients, such as vitamins or minerals, that are beneficial in small amounts.

Disadvantages:

The disadvantages of consuming unhealthy foods regularly are numerous and can have long-term negative effects on your health. Some of the potential negative consequences of consuming these types of foods include:

Weight gain: Consuming too many calories from unhealthy foods can lead to weight gain and obesity, which can increase your risk for numerous health conditions, such as heart disease, diabetes, and certain types of cancer.

Poor nutrient intake: Unhealthy foods are often low in nutrients and high in calories, which can lead to deficiencies in essential vitamins and minerals over time.

Increased risk of chronic diseases: Consuming unhealthy foods regularly can increase your risk of developing chronic diseases, such as heart disease, type 2 diabetes, and certain types of cancer.

Addiction: Some unhealthy foods, such as those high in sugar or salt, can be addictive and lead to cravings and overconsumption.

Poor digestion: Unhealthy foods are often low in fiber and can disrupt your digestive system, leading to issues such as constipation or diarrhea.

is it really possible to avoid processed food from your diet?

While it can be challenging to completely avoid all processed foods, it is possible to significantly reduce your intake of processed foods by making some changes to your diet and lifestyle. Here are some tips that can help:

Choose whole, unprocessed foods: Focus on consuming whole, minimally processed foods such as fruits, vegetables, whole grains, lean proteins, and healthy fats.

Cook at home: Cooking at home allows you to control the ingredients in your meals and avoid highly processed, packaged foods.

Read food labels: When purchasing packaged foods, read the labels and choose products that are minimally processed and have simple, whole food ingredients.

Avoid highly processed snacks: Instead of reaching for highly processed snacks like chips or candy, choose whole foods like fruit, nuts, or hummus with veggies.

Plan ahead: Plan your meals and snacks in advance to ensure that you have healthy, whole food options readily available.

Choose alternatives to processed foods: For example, instead of sugary breakfast cereals, choose oatmeal with fruit and nuts or instead of canned soups, make your own soups from scratch.

While it may not be possible to completely avoid all processed foods, taking these steps can help you significantly reduce your intake and prioritize a healthier diet.

In conclusion

consuming unhealthy foods regularly can have numerous negative consequences on your health. It's important to focus on consuming a balanced diet that includes plenty of fruits, vegetables, lean proteins, and whole grains to ensure that your body receives the nutrients it needs to function properly.

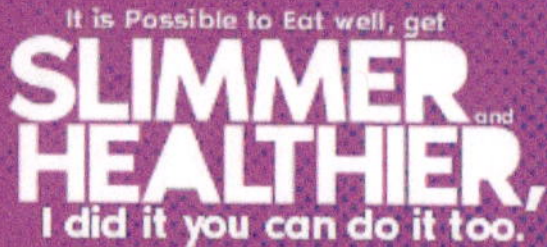

CHAPTER 5

The importance of staying hydrated and consuming enough fluids throughout the day

Staying hydrated and consuming enough fluids throughout the day is crucial for maintaining optimal health and well-being,being hydrated and consuming enough fluids throughout the day is essential for maintaining good health and preventing dehydration-related health issues. It's recommended to drink at least 8 cups (64 ounces) of water per day, but this can vary depending on individual needs, physical activity levels, and climate.

Water plays a crucial role in regulating body temperature. When the body becomes too hot, either due to environmental factors or physical activity, it activates the sweat glands to produce sweat. As sweat evaporates from the skin, it takes heat with it, cooling the body down.

However, if the body is dehydrated, it can struggle to produce enough sweat to regulate body temperature. This can lead to overheating, heat exhaustion, and even heatstroke, which can be life-threatening.

Drinking enough water and staying hydrated can help prevent these issues by ensuring that the body has enough fluids to produce sweat and regulate temperature effectively. In addition, drinking cold water can help lower the body's internal temperature and provide relief on hot days or during intense physical activity.

Staying hydrated is essential for maintaining good health and well-being. Here are some of the ways that hydration helps one stay healthy:

Supports bodily functions: Water is essential for the proper functioning of various bodily systems, including the cardiovascular, digestive, and urinary systems. Staying hydrated ensures that these systems can work optimally and keep the body healthy.

Regulates body temperature: Adequate hydration is necessary for regulating body temperature, which is essential for preventing overheating, heat exhaustion, and heatstroke.

Improves physical performance: Drinking enough water can improve physical performance by increasing endurance, strength, and power. It can also reduce fatigue and improve recovery time after exercise.

Boosts brain function: Proper hydration is essential for maintaining cognitive function, including concentration, memory, and mood. Dehydration can lead to cognitive impairment and negatively impact brain function.

Supports kidney function: Water is essential for maintaining healthy kidney function by flushing out waste and toxins from the body. Without enough water, the kidneys can become stressed and lead to kidney stones and other health issues.

Reduces the risk of infections: Staying hydrated can help reduce the risk of urinary tract infections, as it flushes out bacteria and prevents it from accumulating in the urinary tract.

Improves skin health: Proper hydration can improve skin health by keeping it moisturized and preventing dryness, flakiness, and other skin problems.

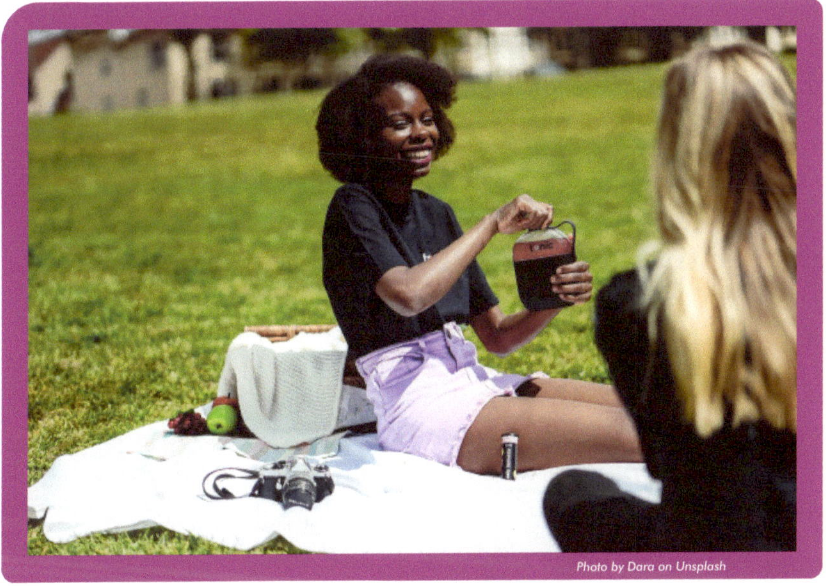
Photo by Dara on Unsplash

Aside from water, there are many other fluids that can help the body stay hydrated, including:

Herbal teas: Herbal teas such as chamomile, peppermint, and ginger tea can help hydrate the body while also providing additional health benefits. These teas are rich in antioxidants and can help reduce inflammation, improve digestion, and promote relaxation.

Coconut water: Coconut water is a natural electrolyte-rich drink that is low in calories and sugar. It can help rehydrate the body after exercise or other physical activities.

Milk: Milk is an excellent source of hydration, as it contains a balance of water, electrolytes, and nutrients such as calcium and vitamin D. Low-fat milk or plant-based milk alternatives such as almond or soy milk are also good options.

Fruit juices: Fruit juices, such as orange or cranberry juice, can be hydrating, but it's important to choose juices with no added sugars and consume them in moderation.

Sports drinks: Sports drinks are designed to provide hydration and replenish electrolytes lost during intense physical activity. However, they can be high in sugar, so it's important to choose low-sugar options and consume them in moderation.

The benefits of staying hydrated with these fluids include maintaining proper hydration levels in the body, supporting bodily functions, improving physical performance, boosting brain function, and reducing the risk of infections. It's important to note that while these fluids can help with hydration, water should still be the primary source of hydration for optimal health and well-being.

Here are some tips for managing a healthy hydrated life daily:

Drink plenty of water: Make sure to drink at least 8 glasses of water a day, and more if you are physically active or in hot weather.

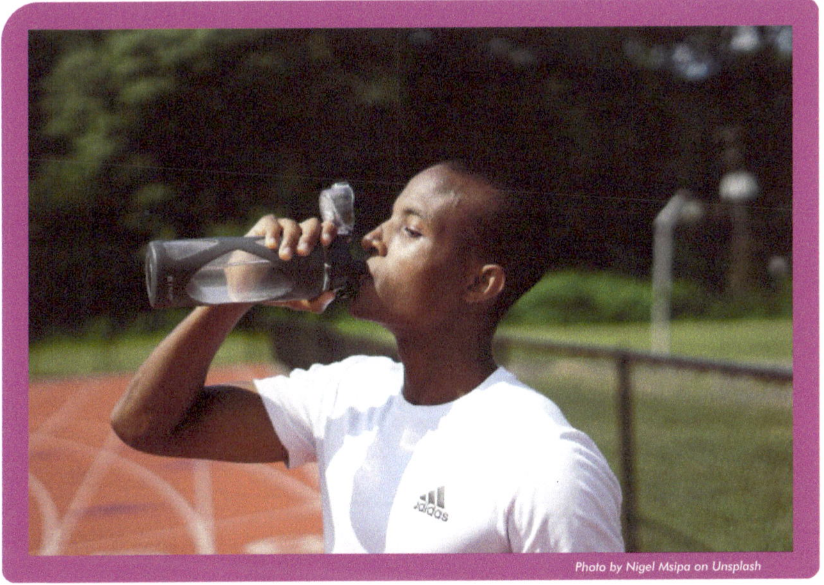

Photo by Nigel Msipa on Unsplash

Carry a reusable water bottle: Keep a reusable water bottle with you at all times so that you can easily stay hydrated throughout the day.

Eat hydrating foods: Incorporate hydrating foods into your diet, such as watermelon, cucumbers, berries, and leafy greens.

Limit caffeine and alcohol: Caffeine and alcohol can be dehydrating, so it's important to limit your intake of these beverages.

Set reminders: Use apps or alarms to remind yourself to drink water throughout the day.

Monitor urine color: Check the color of your urine to ensure that you are properly hydrated. Clear or pale yellow urine indicates proper hydration, while dark yellow or amber-colored urine may indicate dehydration.

Consider electrolyte intake: If you are physically active, consider drinking fluids that contain electrolytes to help replenish the minerals lost through sweat.

Be mindful of hydration during illness: When you are sick, make sure to drink plenty of fluids to prevent dehydration.

In conclusion

hydration is vital for maintaining good health and well-being. Proper hydration helps regulate body temperature, supports bodily functions, improves physical performance, boosts brain function, reduces the risk of infections, and much more. By drinking enough fluids, including water and other hydrating beverages, and following healthy habits to maintain optimal hydration levels, you can help your body function at its best and prevent dehydration-related health problems.

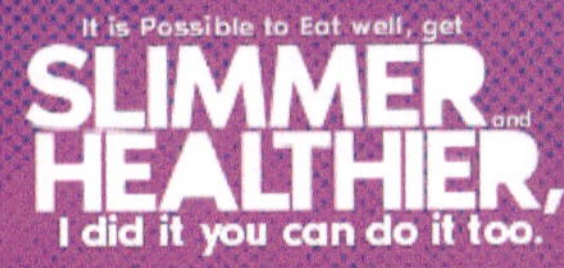

CHAPTER 6

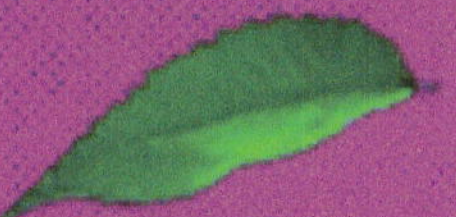

The role of physical activity and exercise in achieving and maintaining a healthy weight

The theory behind physical activity as a means of reducing weight is based on the concept of energy balance. When we consume more calories than we burn through physical activity and other daily activities, the excess calories are stored in the body as fat, leading to weight gain. On the other hand, when we burn more calories than we consume, the body uses stored fat for energy, leading to weight loss.

Physical activity and exercise contribute to weight loss by burning calories and increasing the body's metabolic rate. When we engage in physical activity, the body uses energy to power our muscles and perform the movements. This energy comes from stored carbohydrates and fats in the body. As we continue to exercise, the body burns more calories and taps into stored fat to meet the increased energy demand, leading to weight loss over time.

Additionally, physical activity can help to build muscle mass, which increases the body's metabolic rate and helps to burn calories more efficiently even when at rest. This effect can further contribute to weight loss and weight management.

There are several reasons why many people may fear or avoid engaging in exercise as a means of weight reduction:

Perceived difficulty: Many people believe that exercise is too difficult or requires too much effort, which can be a deterrent to getting started.

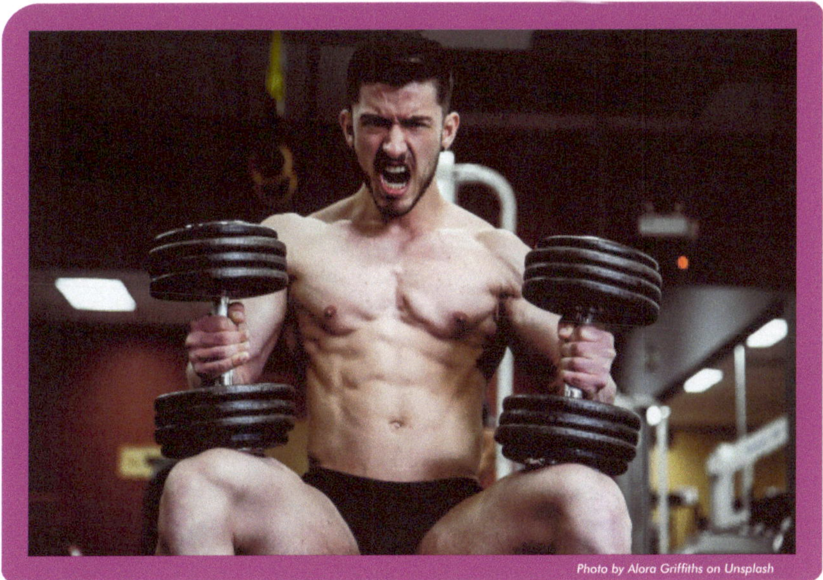

Photo by Alora Griffiths on Unsplash

Time constraints: With busy schedules and competing priorities, finding time for regular exercise can be a challenge for many people.

Lack of motivation: It can be difficult to stay motivated to exercise, particularly if results are not seen immediately.

Fear of injury: Some people may worry about getting injured during exercise, particularly if they are not familiar with proper technique or are starting from a relatively sedentary lifestyle.

Self-consciousness: Some people may feel self-conscious or uncomfortable about exercising in public or in front of others, particularly if they are overweight.

Lack of knowledge: Many people may not know how to get started with an exercise program or may not understand the best types of exercise for weight reduction.

Let me share a personal story of someone who I know that has lost weight from being obese to being fit.

Samantha had struggled with her weight for most of her adult life. She had tried various diets and exercise programs, but nothing seemed to stick. At her heaviest, Samantha weighed 250 pounds, and she knew she needed to make a change.

Samantha started by setting a realistic goal of losing 1-2 pounds per week. She began by tracking her food intake using a mobile app and gradually reducing her calorie intake. She also started walking for 30 minutes every day, gradually increasing her intensity and duration over time.

As Samantha began to see progress, she started to incorporate strength training and other forms of cardio into her routine. She joined a local gym and started attending group fitness classes, which helped her to stay motivated and engaged.

Over the course of a year, Samantha lost 100 pounds and was able to maintain her weight loss by continuing to exercise regularly and make healthy food choices. She found that the key to her success was taking small, sustainable steps towards her goal and finding activities she enjoyed.

Samantha now feels more confident, energized, and healthy than ever before. She no longer feels held back by her weight and has a renewed sense of excitement for life.

Getting motivated to exercise can be a challenging task, especially if you're trying to lose weight. However, regular physical activity is essential to achieving and maintaining a healthy weight. Here are some strategies you can use to stay motivated and committed to your exercise routine:

Set Realistic Goals: Setting realistic and achievable goals can help you stay motivated and committed to your exercise routine. You may want to consider setting specific goals, such as exercising for 30 minutes a day, 5 days a week or losing 1-2 pounds per week.

Find An Exercise You Enjoy: Exercise doesn't have to be a chore. Finding an activity that you enjoy can make it easier to stick to your routine. Whether it's running, swimming, or taking a dance class, there are many ways to get your heart rate up and burn calories.

Keep A Fitness Journal: Keeping track of your progress can be a great motivator. Consider keeping a fitness journal where you can record your exercise routine, weight loss progress, and other achievements. This can help you stay focused and committed to your goals.

Get A Workout Buddy: Exercising with a friend or family

member can make the experience more enjoyable and hold you accountable. Make a plan to work out together on a regular basis, and encourage each other to stay motivated and committed to your routine.

Reward Yourself: Treating yourself to small rewards along the way can help you stay motivated and committed to your exercise routine. Whether it's a new workout outfit, a massage, or a night out with friends, it's important to recognize your hard work and dedication.

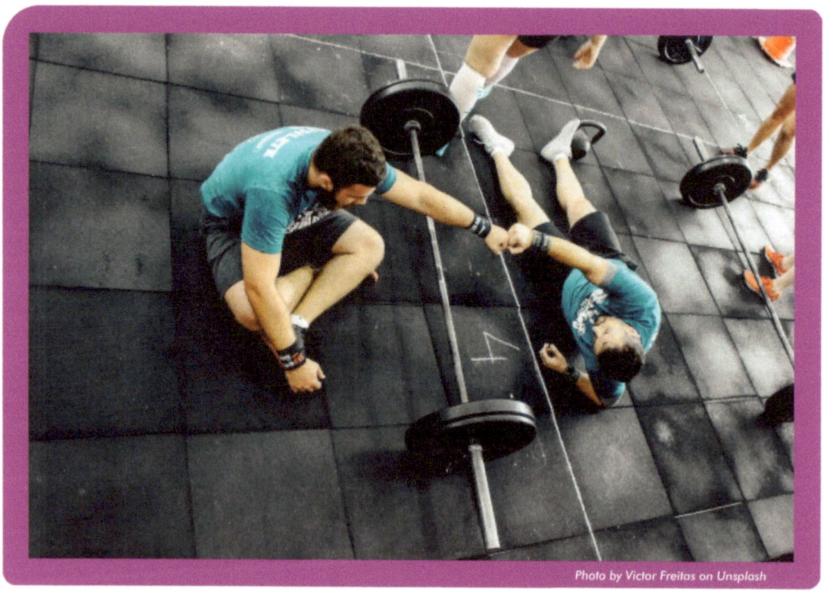

Photo by Victor Freitas on Unsplash

Yes, exercise can help you lose weight. When you exercise, your body burns calories, which can lead to weight loss over time. However, it's important to remember that exercise alone may not be enough to achieve significant weight loss. To lose weight, you need to create a calorie deficit, which means burning more calories than you consume through your diet.

In addition to burning calories, exercise can also help build muscle, which can boost your metabolism and help you burn more calories even when you're not exercising. Exercise can also improve your overall health and well-being, reducing your risk of chronic diseases such as heart disease, diabetes, and cancer.

It's important to note that exercise should be combined with a healthy diet for effective weight loss. Eating a balanced diet with plenty of fruits, vegetables, lean protein, and whole grains can provide the nutrients your body needs to fuel your workouts and support weight loss.

In conclusion

Exercise can help you lose weight, but it should be combined with a healthy diet for best results. By creating a calorie deficit through exercise and diet, you can achieve and maintain a healthy weight while improving your overall health and well-being.

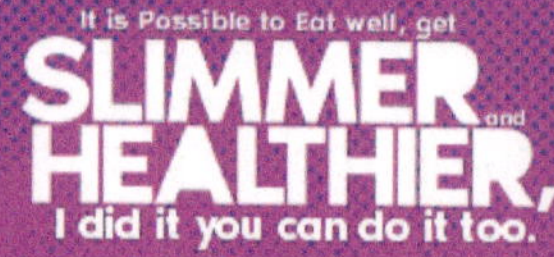

CHAPTER 7

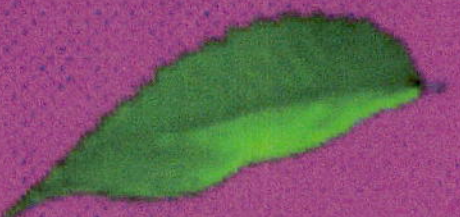

The potential benefits of Incorporating healthy fats into the diet, such as those found in nuts, seeds, and fatty fish

Dietary fat often gets a bad reputation, but the truth is, not all fats are created equal. In fact, certain types of fats are considered "healthy" fats that provide substantial health benefits. These healthy fats play numerous important roles in the body when consumed in recommended amounts and appropriate balance.

This chapter provides an extensive look at the different types of beneficial fats, why they are important for overall wellbeing, and how incorporating more healthy fats into your diet can impart both short-term and long-lasting advantages.

Types of Healthy Fats

There are several categories of fats considered healthy when consumed in moderation:

Monounsaturated Fatty Acids:
Like olive, peanut, safflower, sesame, and canola oils. Also found in avocados, nuts, and seeds.

Polyunsaturated Fatty Acids:
Omega-3 fatty acids - Found in fatty fish, walnuts, flaxseed, chia seeds.

Omega-6 fatty acids - Found in vegetable oils, nuts and seeds.

Medium Chain Triglycerides:
Found in coconut oil, palm oil, and dairy products.

The common factor between all these healthy fats is that they mainly consist of monounsaturated or polyunsaturated fatty acids with a liquid consistency at room temperature. The exceptions are medium chain triglycerides, which maintain liquid form regardless of temperature due to their smaller structure.

Benefits for Heart Health

Various epidemiological studies have found diets higher in monounsaturated and polyunsaturated fats correlate with lower rates of cardiovascular disease and mortality compared to diets higher in saturated fats or trans fats.

In particular, replacing dietary saturated fats with unsaturated fats has been shown to:

- Lower low-density lipoprotein (LDL or "bad") cholesterol
- Raise high-density lipoprotein (HDL or "good") cholesterol
- Improve endothelial function and arterial flexibility
- Lower blood pressure
- Reduce inflammation
- Lower risk of developing atherosclerosis

These effects promote overall cardiovascular health and reduce risk factors for several common heart conditions. The American Heart Association recommends getting 5-10% of total calories from omega-6 oils and eating at least two 3.5 oz servings of fatty fish per week for optimal heart health.

Effects on Cholesterol Profile

As mentioned, increasing specific healthy fats while limiting saturated and trans fats has clinically demonstrated effects of lowering LDL cholesterol while raising HDL cholesterol.

LDL cholesterol accumulates in arteries and heightens risk for heart attack and stroke. HDL cholesterol has antioxidant effects and is considered protective by transporting cholesterol from arteries back to the liver for elimination. The balance between these two types of cholesterol profiles is a key predictor of cardiovascular disease progression.

According to a meta-analysis in the American Journal of Clinical Nutrition, exchanging 1% of daily caloric intake from saturated fats to an isocaloric amount of polyunsaturated fats lowers LDL cholesterol by ~2 mg/dL while raising HDL by ~0.5 mg/dL. Small consistent changes adding up over months/years can shift patients from high-risk to optimal cholesterol profiles.

Effects on Inflammation

Chronic inflammation is known as a key driver behind

numerous modern health conditions ranging from cardiovascular disease to autoimmune disorders, neurocognitive decline, and cancers.

Higher intakes of anti-inflammatory omega-3s from fatty fish, nuts and seeds helps balance out pro-inflammatory omega-6 fatty acids to reduce systemic inflammation. Medium chain triglycerides found in coconut oil also have anti-inflammatory properties according to recent research.

Replacing dietary arachidonic acid, an omega-6 fatty acid that can be pro-inflammatory, with anti-inflammatory eicosapentaenoic acid (EPA) and docosahexaenoic acid (DHA) from fatty fish has clinically demonstrated reductions in circulating inflammatory biomarkers like TNF-a, IL-6, and CRP.

Importance for Brain Health

The long-chain omega-3 fatty acids EPA and DHA play imperative roles in optimal nervous system functioning at all stages of life. These polyunsaturated fats:

Are highly concentrated in brain cell membranes

Help form nerve cell insulation that allows efficient neurotransmission

- Reduce neuroinflammation

- Promote neural plasticity

- Support neuron resilience

As a result, adequate intake of EPA and DHA has been associated with:

- Sharper memory and improved learning capacity
- Slower cognitive decline
- Reduced risk of dementia
- Better mental health with lower rates of depression/anxiety symptoms

During fetal development, maternal intake of omega-3s has even been linked to superior vision, intelligence, and motor skills in offspring. Many experts recommend at least 250–500 mg/day of combined EPA and DHA.

Other Health Benefits

In addition to cardiovascular and brain benefits, diets higher in various healthy fats provide a spectrum of other evidence-based health advantages:

- Increased satiety after meals & improved weight control
- Reduction in risk for metabolic syndrome and type 2 diabetes
- Potential anti-cancer activity and slower cancer progression
- Lower systemic inflammation benefits for autoimmune disorders
- Improved bone mineral density
- Healthier skin, hair, and nails
- Better vision health
- Enhanced strength and athletic performance

There are even studies linking higher monounsaturated fat intake to increased life expectancy. Replacing dietary carbohydrates with any type of fat is associated with decreased mortality risk, but monounsaturated fats like olive oil confer the greatest benefits.

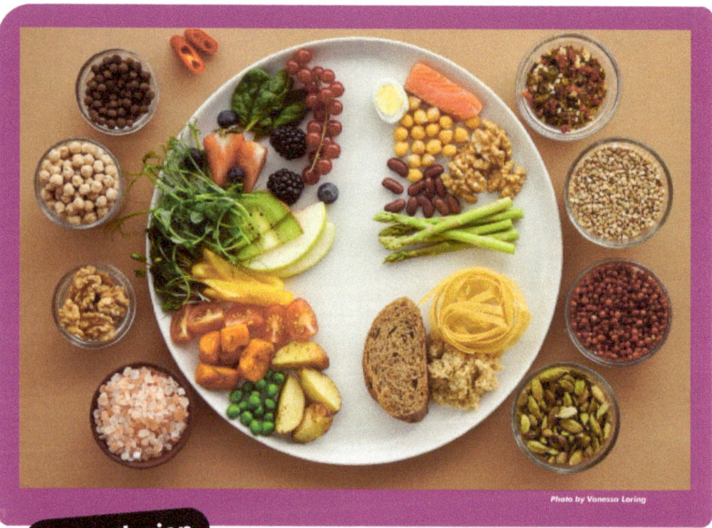

Photo by Vanessa Loring

In conclusion

Despite outdated misconceptions about all fats equally contributing to poor health, the latest science clearly demonstrates incorporating more healthy monounsaturated, polyunsaturated, and medium chain triglyceride fats provides measurable advantages for nearly every aspect of wellness. From the brain to the heart, cells throughout the body thrive when supplied with regular intake of beneficial fats from nutritious whole food sources. An individualized nutrition plan higher in foods like olive oil, nuts, seeds, avocados and fatty fish is exceedingly likely to lead to better health and longevity.

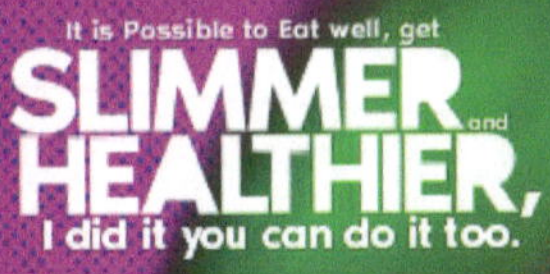

CHAPTER 8

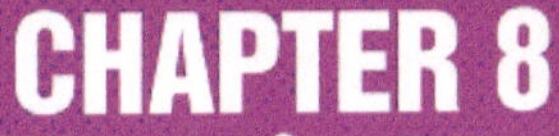

Strategies for managing cravings and overcoming obstacles to eating well

For many people trying to improve their dietary habits, inconvenient cravings and external obstacles present consistent challenges on the path towards healthier eating. Difficulty staying on track can subsequently lead to frustration, self-criticism, and abandoning positive changes altogether when willpower wears thin.

However, by better understanding the science behind cravings along with proven techniques to outsmart common pitfalls, you can take control when tempting urges strike and circumvent situations sabotaging your eating goals. This chapter provides guidance on easing cravings, dodging triggers, creating accountability, keeping perspective, and maintaining motivation to overcome the inevitable hurdles en route to genuine, lasting positive changes.

Why Cravings Happen

In many cases, food cravings stem from biological shifts or nutritional shortcomings signaling the body to seek out specific nutrients. For instance, cravings for sweets can arise from low serotonin levels, chocolate from magnesium deficiencies, and salty foods from mineral imbalances or adrenal fatigue.

Cravings can also be emotional or psychological in origin, triggered by connections formed in the brain's reward center linking certain feelings to particular foods. Things like stress, boredom, anxiety, loneliness and even happiness or celebration can set off cravings entwined with these emotions.

Understanding your personal common craving triggers can help you better navigate and defuse those challenging moments when only one food will do.

Strategies to Curb Cravings

When an intense urge strikes for chocolate, chips or other temptation foods, having reliable techniques in your back pocket makes maintaining willpower much more feasible. Here are methods to calm cravings effectively:

Distract - Shift your focus to something enjoyable yet unrelated to food, like calling a friend or hobby activity for 10-15 minutes until the intensity passes.

Delay - Tell yourself you can have the food later if the craving persists rather than denying completely, which alleviates the psychological tug-of-war. Often after postponing the urge fades.

Distance - Physically move away from the triggering environment by stepping outdoors or leaving the kitchen to create space from the temptation.

Drink - Hydration levels influence satiety signals. Pour a glass of water with lemon and drink slowly. You may have misinterpreted thirst cues as food urges.

Breathe - Stress exacerbates cravings. Try square breathing: inhale for 4 counts, hold for 4 counts, exhale for 4 counts.

Repeat until calm.

Swap - Pick a healthier substitute providing satisfaction with more nutrients and fewer empty calories.

Dodging Obstacle Course Traps

In addition to spontaneous cravings, aspects of daily life like demanding work hours, social pressures and exposure to endless food availability can also derail positive nutrition habits. Here are tips to sidestep common pitfalls:

Meal Prep - Pack healthy grab-and-go snacks and cook bulk servings of nutritious dishes twice per week to always have wholesome options on hand.

Set Limits - Practice saying "no" to offers of treats in the office or rich restaurant dishes with confidence rather than feeling deprived.

Avoid Tempting Aisles - Speed shop mostly around the periphery of grocery stores where whole foods like produce and proteins are sold to limit exposure to processed snacks.

Bring Your Own - Maintain clean eating standards at parties or holidays by contributing a healthy plant-based dish so you're guaranteed satisfying options.

Seek Support - Connect with coworkers or join an online

community trying to improve similar eating habits for camaraderie through challenges.

Learn Triggers - Keep a food journal tracking mood before and after eating certain items to identify personal pitfall foods or emotions derailing you. Understanding these relationships is key to preventing missteps.

Cultivating Accountability and Motivation

In addition to practical strategies for navigating cravings and barriers in the moment, establishing structural accountability and motivation systems dramatically improves your likelihood of maintaining healthy changes long-term when you're lacking willpower. Consider leveraging tools like the following:

Health Coaching - Working with a qualified health coach provides professional guidance, resources, accountability check-ins and emotional support which all reinforce positive changes.

Enlist a Partner - Ask a friend with similar goals to check in weekly and cheer each other's small wins while troubleshooting hurdles that arise together.

Food Journaling - Recording all food and drink consumed in an app along with hunger, emotions and energy levels before/after eating keeps you conscious of progress and slip-ups.

Focus on Wins -Post motivational reminders of bigger reasons for eating well or celebrate small milestones like successful weeklong avoidance of vending machine snacks.

Consider Supplements - In some cases, targeted nutritional supplements can help curb cravings by restoring deficiencies driving certain cravings. Speak to a registered dietitian about options.

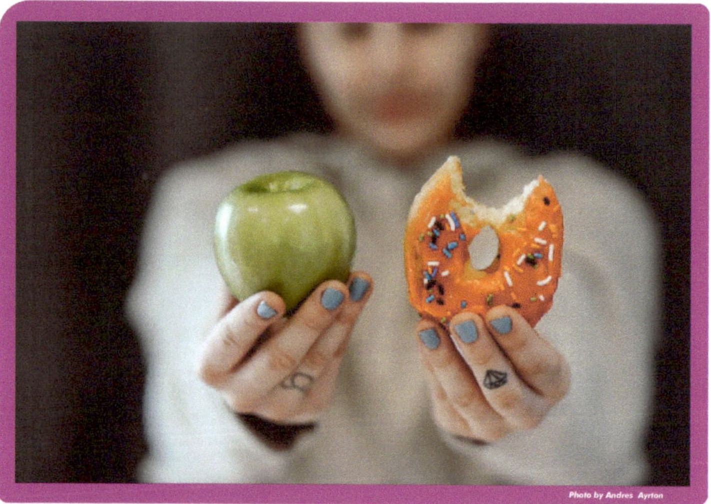

In conclusion

Instead of an all-or-nothing battle for perfection with eating, take the pressure off yourself by accepting slip-ups as inevitable while aiming gently for progress over perfection. Arm yourself with craving coping strategies for the challenging moments while establishing motivational systems and social support to smooth the path towards genuine healthier eating habits in the long run. With some thoughtful planning and self-compassion, overcoming those pesky cravings is within your reach.

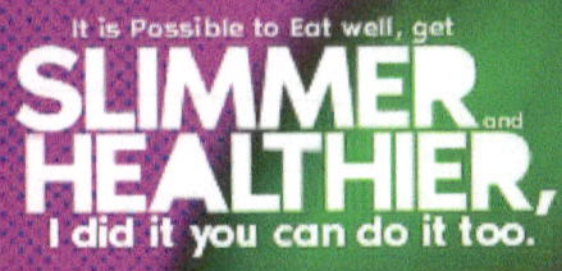

CHAPTER 9

The importance of getting enough sleep and managing stress for overall health and weight management

An often overlooked element in developing a healthy lifestyle is the vital role of two resource management systems that exert enormous influence over physical, mental, and emotional wellbeing - sleep and stress levels. Getting ample, high-quality sleep and keeping stress within healthy parameters provides a strong foundation upon which all other dimensions of wellness depend.

The Effects of Inadequate Sleep

Although people still assume losing sleep is a relatively harmless experience in modern life, science has demonstrated the deep ramifications that chronic sleep deprivation can induce over time. Lacking just 1-2 hours of recommended sleep (7-9 hours/night) for days/weeks in a row is enough to impair key systems to an extent equivalent to intoxication due to alcohol. Here are some ways insufficient sleep drags health down in interconnected ripple effects:

Mental Effects - Poor memory, slower mental processing, lack of alertness, concentration impairment

Hormone Effects - Disrupted balance between leptin/ghrelin increasing hunger so overeating more common

Weight Effects - More fat storage with reduced ability to lose excess weight due to metabolic effects

Immune Effects - Reduced natural killer cells and infection-fighting antibodies making frequent illness more likely

Mood Effects - Higher sensitivity to stress, inability to regulate emotions as well, increased anxiety/depression

Energy Effects - Reliance on stress hormones for alertness instead of truly restorative energy through sleep

This sets off a distressing cycle - without understanding sleep deprivation as the root cause driving physical and emotional dysfunction, symptomatic issues themselves only serve to perpetuate worsening sleep due to worry or discomfort.

Strategies to Improve Sleep Quality

To achieve healthy, consistent sleep, a sleep hygiene routine removing sleep obstacles is critical. These best practices prime mind and body for smooth initiation, maintenance, and progression of sleep cycles throughout the night:

Follow a regular sleep-wake schedule, even weekends

Develop relaxing pre-bedtime rituals like warm baths, reading

Remove electronics from the bedroom

Block out light/noise disturbances

Address pain, anxiety, frequent urination issues hindering sleep

Limit alcohol as it impairs sleep quality later at night

Tracking sleep quality will also help diagnose issues preventing you from feeling well-rested. If problems persist despite behavioral adjustments, speak to your doctor as there are numerous medical conditions potentially at play.

The Science of Stress

Just as deprivation of sleep takes an undercover toll across health parameters, the consequences of unmanaged stress also disrupt homeostasis. While our primitive ancestors evolved a "fight-or-flight response" using stress hormones like adrenaline and cortisol to ensure survival in times of danger, most of today's threats are psychological rather than life-threatening. The outdated yet hardwired intensity of this response then takes a progressive toll over time without relief through genuine relaxation to turn it off.

The stress hormone cortisol is especially damaging when chronically elevated due to links with obesity, hypertension, insulin resistance, reproductive dysfunction, digestive issues and mental illnesses through inflammatory effects and interference of other essential hormones in the body. Managing stress effectively is therefore critical to prevent far-reaching harm to wellbeing.

Techniques to Counter Stress

To keep stress overload from sinking health, a multi-tiered approach covering physical, mental, and lifestyle angles is needed to address both the symptoms and root causes of excess strain:

Physical Approaches:

- Daily movement - aerobics, strength training - metabolizes stress chemicals
- Sufficient sleep - prevents compounding impact of stress reactions through fatigue
- Yoga, stretching, massage - soothes nervous system with deep muscular relaxation

Mental Approaches:

- Meditation - reduces anxiety and emotional overwhelm
- Mindset shifts - adjust unrealistic expectations and perfectionist tendencies
- Gratitude practices - counterbrain wired to fixate disproportionately on negative
- Emotional healing - address buried issues now manifesting as chronic stress through therapy

Lifestyle Approaches:

- Simplify obligations - reduce unnecessary hurry and pressure demands of modern life

- Meaning and purpose - connect to values beyond pressured productivity
- Work-life balance - set boundaries and take time off to rejuvenate
- Build nurturing relationships - social support through stress improves coping ability

Once disrupting stress reactions themselves, the above foundations better support making lasting positive changes even in difficult times.

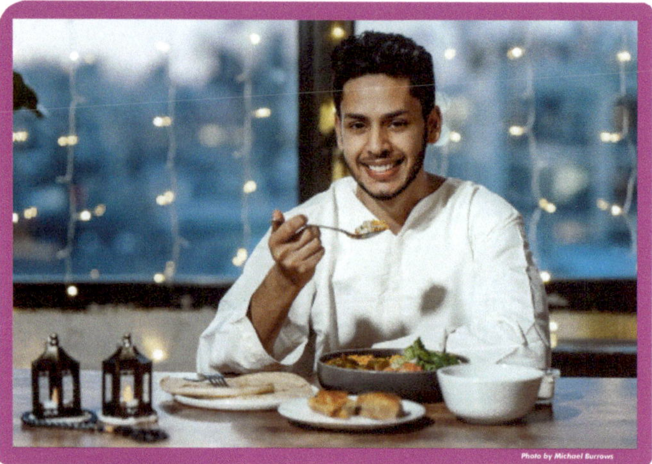

In conclusion

Managing sleep and stress well ripples out to every corner of health due to the direct regulatory influence these interconnected systems exert over involuntary body processes. By understanding their scientifically validated importance and learning techniques to support these critical functions effectively, the path to overall wellbeing and an optimized environment for healthy changes becomes infinitely more achievable. The time and focus dedicated to build up sleep and dial down stress provides enormous dividends across lifetime health and happiness.

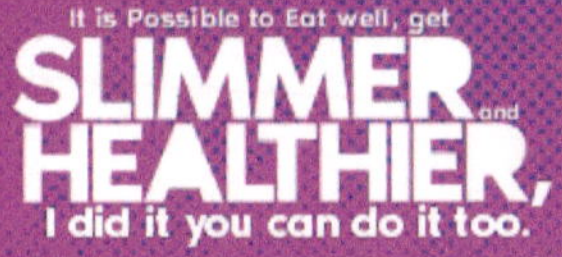

CHAPTER 10

The role of support from friends, family, and healthcare professionals in achieving and maintaining a healthy weight.

When aspiring to achieve ambitious goals like meaningful weight loss followed by lifelong maintenance of a healthy body, it's easy to assume the journey ahead rests primarily on your own shoulders. However, decades of psychological and sociological research reveals we humans rely heavily on community connections and supportive relationships to either enable or thwart major lifestyle changes.

Given obesity now impacts over 40% of the American adult population with associated illness killing tens of thousands annually, transforming dysfunctional eating habits and sedentary norms requires social motivation as a catalyst driving sustainable change. This chapter explains why actively building a circle of positive support across domains of friends, family, and specialized health experts dramatically empowers the weight loss process rather than traversing the rocky road alone.

Friends - The Power of Camaraderie

Casual acquaintances hold minimal influence over motivations behind bettering health, but studies find closer friend groups directly impact mindsets and behaviors tied to weight through peer pressure effects. Whether for better or worse depends greatly on the norms and priorities in a given social circle.

Some communities tacitly enable unhealthy lifestyle factors like drinking, chronic stress, disordered eating habits, and couch potato leisure time reinforcing excess weight gain. You may require expanding social circles or better curating existing friends to find those willing to embark on reciprocal journey towards wellness together.

The beauty of shared experience is normalizing struggles while doubling joy by having a comrade with whom to celebrate victories, exchange ideas, grieve setbacks, and foster accountability. In short, finding your "health tribe" greases wheels of change.

Family - The Power of Roots

Family units established during childhood imprint social norms and mindsets early in life, sowing seeds for challenges like poor body image, chronic dieting, and weight cycling years down the road. Research shows parents overweight or obsessive regarding food/weight anchors similar attitudes in children through modeling.

Whether raised in a household where emotional support got replaced with piles of pasta or fast food was the only affordable dinner option nightly, upending these familial patterns lodged deep in psyche remains challenging but essential work for securing health long-term.

If your family of origin does not currently support establishing new nutritious cooking traditions, moving more, loving your body, and releasing outdated assumptions about diets or weight equaling human value, you may need to limit time with them initially when getting unstuck from ruts. Limiting exposure to naysayers and unhealthy dynamics lifts burden so your wingspan for change can expand.

Doctors - The Power of Expertise

When it comes to solving complex health conditions, credentialed medical and allied health practitioners provide immense value for the expertise gleaned through years of specialized education and hands-on patient experience.

Yet with weight management specifically, traditional doctors often lack training in key realms like nutrition science, psychology of disordered eating, fitness programming, sleep hygiene, hormone balancing, and stress management that address obstacles preventing sustainable change.

Seeking out a specialized bariatric doctor or comprehensive weight management clinic housing a coordinated team of professionals across specialties ensures personalized guidance tackling all dimensions of your struggles is available conveniently under one roof.

Having lab testing uncover potential metabolic or hormonal imbalances, unconditional counseling unearthing root causes of emotional eating tendencies, and an on-demand dietician poring over food logs to calibrate macro goals to your lifestyle proves well worth the investment for solving the puzzle of weight loss resistance once and for all.

successful long term weight management requires a Judgment-free team supporting mind, body and emotional wellbeing. Compassionate yet firm accountability partners, encouraging cheerleaders lifting your spirits, veteran mentors who guide the process, and healthcare experts informed by science collectively help make vision reality - one small lifelong change at a time. With this trusty support squad behind you, the winds of change gaining momentum start feeling exciting rather than intimidating.

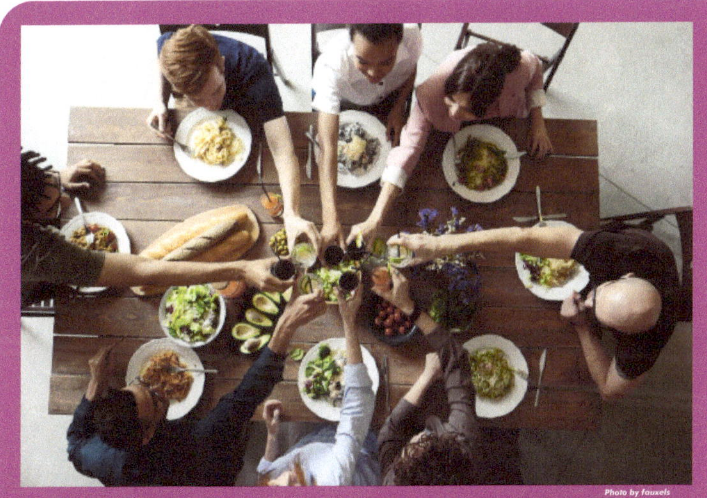

Photo by fauxels

In conclusion

Ultimately the team of supporters cheering you on shapes success reaching finish line of your healthier body goals. Curating a circle of friends modeling positive habits, finding the right medical experts to troubleshoot barriers, and either establishing or limiting family ties to foster self-care in place of self-sabotage stacks conditions for victory in your favor. With this A-team surrounding you on all sides, the winds of change behind your sails start feeling exciting rather than intimidating. Your brighter future awaits!

It is Possible to Eat well, get
SLIMMER and HEALTHIER,
I did it you can do it too.

SUMMARY

After struggling with weight for years and trying every fad diet under the sun with little long-term success, i finally realized we needed to take a holistic lifestyle approach focused on overall wellness rather than just quick weight loss. This book shares the journey of transforming your eating habits, fitness routine, stress management, and relationship with our bodies to finally achieve sustainable weight loss and better health.

Key highlights of the book include:

- The step-by-step process of identifying and overcoming past triggers causing overeating and sedentary behaviors

-

- Developing a healthy, balanced diet tailored to personal preferences that supports weight goals

-

- Incorporating regular exercise with realistic fitness plans for all levels

-

- The importance of a reliable support network for motivation and accountability

-

- Techniques for cultivating more self-compassion and positive body image

-

- Setting small sustainable goals and celebrating mini-milestones along the way

- Relapsing occasionally without catastrophic thinking by getting back on track

-

- Maintenance plans and habits to stick with long after reaching goal weight

This inspiring personal success story aims to motivate readers stuck in similar ruts that achieving better health, slimmer bodies, and balanced lifestyles is within anyone's reach through incremental changes. If ican completely transform long-standing habits in sustainable ways, you can too!

It is Possible to Eat well, get
SLIMMER and
HEALTHIER,
I did it you can do it too.

BOOK BY
BLESSED WOWPLUS
HEALTH NUTRIONIST

www.ingramcontent.com/pod-product-compliance
Lightning Source LLC
Chambersburg PA
CBHW040228240726
48664CB00001B/53